DR. BARBARA CURE FOR HIGH BLOOD PRESSURE

Discover Dr. Barbara Natural Remedies; Combat High Blood Pressure Naturally With Proven Holistic Methods For A Healthier Life

Felipe Carmen

Table of Contents

CHAPTER ONE 5

Introduction to Dr. Barbara's Holistic Approach to Managing High Blood Pressure with Herbs 5

Understanding High Blood Pressure: 6

Dr. Barbara's Holistic Approach: 6

The Role of Herbs in Managing High Blood Pressure: 6

Mechanisms of Action of Herbs: 7

Practical Guidelines for Using Herbs: 8

Conclusion: 9

CHAPTER TWO 9

Understanding High Blood Pressure: Dr. Barbara's Insights into the Condition and Its Impact on Health 9

The Basics of High Blood Pressure: 10

Understanding Blood Pressure Readings: 10

The Impact of High Blood Pressure on Health: 10

Dr. Barbara's Insights into Hypertension: 11

Addressing Root Causes: 11

The Role of Herbs in Managing Hypertension: 12

Conclusion: 12

CHAPTER THREE 13

The Healing Power of Herbs: How Herbal Remedies Can Support Blood Pressure Regulation 13

Understanding Herbal Medicine: 14

Herbs for Blood Pressure Regulation: 14

Mechanisms of Action: 15

Integration into a Holistic Approach: 16

CHAPTER FOUR 17

Preparing for Your Healing Journey: Setting Goals and Gathering Herbal Ingredients 17

Setting Clear Goals: 18

Selecting Herbal Ingredients: 19

Gathering Essential Ingredients: 20

CHAPTER FIVE 22

Selecting the Right Herbs: Dr. Barbara's Recommended Ingredients for Managing High Blood Pressure 22

CHAPTER SIX 27

Crafting Healing Recipes: Herbal Formulas and Teas Designed to Lower Blood Pressure Naturally 27

Herbal Formula for Blood Pressure Regulation: 27

Tips for Crafting Healing Recipes: 30

CHAPTER SEVEN 31

Incorporating Additional Lifestyle Changes: Enhancing the Effectiveness of Herbal Treatment 31

CHAPTER EIGHT..36

Navigating Challenges: Tips for Adjusting to Herbal Remedies and Monitoring Blood Pressure Levels 36

CHAPTER NINE 40

Success Stories: Real-Life Accounts of Individuals Who Have Improved Their High Blood Pressure Through Herbal Treatment 40

CHAPTER TEN 44

Beyond Herbal Remedies: Integrating Dr. Barbara's Principles for Long-Term Blood Pressure Management and Overall Health 44

BONUS: SOME HERBAL REMEDIES TO KNOW 48

THE END...83

COPYRIGHT © 2023

CHAPTER ONE

Introduction to Dr. Barbara's Holistic Approach to Managing High Blood Pressure with Herbs

In contemporary healthcare, the holistic approach to managing high blood pressure (hypertension) has gained significant attention. It emphasizes treating the individual as a whole, addressing not just the symptoms but also the underlying causes and contributing factors. Dr. Barbara, a renowned herbalist and holistic health practitioner, has developed a comprehensive approach to managing high blood pressure using herbs. In this detailed exploration, we will delve into the principles of Dr. Barbara's holistic approach, the effectiveness of herbs in managing hypertension, the mechanisms of action of these herbs, and practical guidelines for their usage.

Understanding High Blood Pressure:

Before delving into Dr. Barbara's holistic approach, it's crucial to understand high blood pressure and its implications. High blood pressure occurs when the force of blood against the artery walls is consistently too high. This condition, if left untreated, can lead to serious health complications such as heart disease, stroke, and kidney failure. Both genetic and lifestyle factors contribute to the development of hypertension, including diet, physical inactivity, stress, and obesity.

Dr. Barbara's Holistic Approach:

Dr. Barbara's holistic approach to managing high blood pressure integrates various modalities, including herbal medicine, nutrition, lifestyle modifications, and stress management techniques. Unlike conventional medicine, which often focuses solely on medications to lower blood pressure, Dr. Barbara's approach recognizes the interconnectedness of the body systems and aims to restore balance and harmony.

The Role of Herbs in Managing High Blood Pressure:

Herbal medicine has been used for centuries in the treatment of various ailments, including hypertension. Certain herbs possess properties that help regulate blood pressure levels by dilating blood vessels, reducing inflammation, and promoting relaxation. Dr. Barbara carefully selects herbs based on their efficacy and safety profiles, ensuring optimal results with minimal side effects.

Mechanisms of Action of Herbs:

Herbs exert their antihypertensive effects through various mechanisms, including:

1. **Vasodilation:** Certain herbs, such as hawthorn (Crataegus spp.) and garlic (Allium sativum), contain compounds that help relax blood vessels, thereby reducing peripheral resistance and lowering blood pressure.

2. **Diuretic Action:** Herbs like dandelion (Taraxacum officinale) and parsley (Petroselinum crispum) have diuretic properties, promoting the excretion of excess fluid and sodium from the body, which can help lower blood pressure.

3. **Antioxidant Activity:** Many herbs are rich in antioxidants, such as flavonoids and polyphenols, which help protect blood vessels from oxidative damage and inflammation, contributing to overall cardiovascular health.

4. **Stress Reduction:** Adaptogenic herbs like ashwagandha (Withaniasomnifera) and holy basil (Ocimum sanctum) help the body adapt to stress and promote relaxation, which can indirectly lower blood pressure by reducing stress hormone levels.

Practical Guidelines for Using Herbs:

When incorporating herbs into a holistic approach for managing high blood pressure, it's essential to consider the following guidelines:

1. **Consultation with a Qualified Practitioner:** Before starting any herbal regimen, consult with a qualified herbalist or healthcare provider, especially if you're currently taking medications or have underlying health conditions.

2. **Individualized Treatment:** Dr. Barbara emphasizes the importance of personalized treatment plans tailored to each

individual's unique constitution, health history, and lifestyle factors.

3. **Quality and Safety:** Choose high-quality herbs from reputable sources to ensure purity, potency, and safety. Avoid herbs that may interact with medications or exacerbate existing health conditions.

4. **Consistency and Patience:** Herbal medicine often requires consistent use over time to yield noticeable results. Be patient and allow sufficient time for the herbs to exert their therapeutic effects.

5. **Lifestyle Modifications:** In conjunction with herbal therapy, adopt healthy lifestyle habits such as a balanced diet, regular exercise, stress management techniques, and adequate sleep to optimize blood pressure control.

Conclusion:

Dr. Barbara's holistic approach to managing high blood pressure with herbs offers a comprehensive and individualized alternative to conventional medication-focused treatments. By addressing the root causes of hypertension and promoting overall health and well-being, this approach empowers individuals to take an active role in managing their blood pressure naturally. With careful guidance from qualified practitioners and adherence to lifestyle modifications, herbal medicine can serve as a valuable adjunct or alternative therapy in the management of hypertension.

CHAPTER TWO

Understanding High Blood Pressure: Dr. Barbara's Insights into the Condition and Its Impact on Health

High blood pressure, also known as hypertension, is a common cardiovascular condition characterized by elevated pressure in the arteries. Dr. Barbara, a holistic health practitioner, provides valuable insights into this condition, its underlying mechanisms, and its impact on overall health.

The Basics of High Blood Pressure:

At its core, high blood pressure refers to the force exerted by blood against the walls of the arteries. This force is influenced by the amount of blood pumped by the heart and the resistance to blood flow in the arteries. When this pressure remains consistently elevated over time, it can damage the blood vessels and lead to serious health complications.

Understanding Blood Pressure Readings:

Blood pressure readings consist of two numbers: systolic and diastolic. Systolic pressure represents the force exerted by the blood against the artery walls when the heart contracts, while diastolic pressure reflects the pressure when the heart is at rest between beats. Normal blood pressure is typically considered to be around 120/80 mmHg. However, readings above this range may indicate prehypertension or hypertension, depending on the severity.

The Impact of High Blood Pressure on Health:

High blood pressure is often referred to as the "silent killer" because it usually presents with no symptoms in its early stages. However, if left untreated, it can significantly increase the risk of various health complications, including:

1. **Heart Disease:** Hypertension can strain the heart muscles, leading to conditions such as coronary artery disease, heart attack, and heart failure.

2. **Stroke:** Elevated blood pressure can damage the blood vessels in the brain, increasing the risk of stroke, which occurs when blood flow to the brain is disrupted.

3. **Kidney Damage:** The kidneys play a crucial role in regulating blood pressure. Chronic hypertension can impair kidney function and increase the risk of kidney disease or failure.

4. **Vision Loss:** High blood pressure can damage the blood vessels in the eyes, leading to vision problems and, in severe cases, vision loss.

5. **Peripheral Artery Disease:** Reduced blood flow to the limbs due to narrowed or blocked arteries can result in peripheral artery disease, causing pain, numbness, and impaired wound healing.

Dr. Barbara's Insights into Hypertension:

Dr. Barbara emphasizes a holistic understanding of hypertension, considering not only the physiological factors but also the underlying emotional, mental, and environmental influences. She recognizes that hypertension is often a multifactorial condition influenced by genetics, lifestyle choices, stress, diet, and environmental factors.

Addressing Root Causes:

Rather than simply treating the symptoms of high blood pressure with medications, Dr. Barbara advocates for identifying and addressing the root causes of hypertension. This may involve lifestyle modifications, stress management techniques, dietary changes, and holistic therapies aimed at restoring balance and optimizing overall health.

The Role of Herbs in Managing Hypertension:

Dr. Barbara integrates herbal medicine into her approach to managing hypertension, leveraging the therapeutic properties of various herbs to support cardiovascular health. Herbs such as hawthorn, garlic, dandelion, and parsley have been traditionally used for their antihypertensive effects, helping to regulate blood pressure levels naturally.

Conclusion:

Dr. Barbara's insights into high blood pressure provide a comprehensive understanding of this prevalent cardiovascular condition and its impact on health. By recognizing the interconnectedness of physiological, emotional, and environmental factors, she emphasizes a holistic approach to managing hypertension. Through lifestyle modifications, stress management, dietary interventions, and the strategic use of herbal medicine, individuals can take proactive steps to control their blood pressure and promote long-term cardiovascular health.

CHAPTER THREE

The Healing Power of Herbs: How Herbal Remedies Can Support Blood Pressure Regulation

Herbal remedies have been used for centuries to promote health and alleviate various ailments, including high blood pressure (hypertension). Dr. Barbara, a holistic health practitioner, recognizes the healing potential of herbs in supporting blood pressure regulation. In this exploration, we delve into the mechanisms by which herbal remedies exert their therapeutic effects on hypertension and how they can be integrated into a holistic approach to health and wellness.

Understanding Herbal Medicine:

Herbal medicine, also known as phytotherapy, involves the use of plants and plant extracts to prevent and treat health conditions. Herbs contain a diverse array of bioactive compounds, including flavonoids, alkaloids, and polyphenols, which contribute to their medicinal properties. When used appropriately, herbal remedies can offer gentle yet effective support for various health concerns, including hypertension.

Herbs for Blood Pressure Regulation:

Several herbs have demonstrated promising effects in supporting blood pressure regulation. These herbs work through various mechanisms to help lower blood pressure and promote cardiovascular health. Some of the key herbs commonly used for this purpose include:

1. **Hawthorn (Crataegus spp.):** Hawthorn berries and leaves are rich in flavonoids and procyanidins, which have vasodilatory effects, helping to relax and dilate blood vessels. This can lead to improved blood flow and reduced blood pressure levels.

2. **Garlic (Allium sativum):** Garlic contains sulfur compounds such as allicin, which have been shown to have hypotensive properties. Garlic supplementation may help lower both systolic and diastolic blood pressure by promoting vasodilation and reducing peripheral resistance.

3. **Hibiscus (Hibiscus sabdariffa):** Hibiscus tea is rich in antioxidants, including anthocyanins and polyphenols, which have been linked to reductions in blood pressure. Hibiscus may also have diuretic effects, promoting the excretion of excess fluid and sodium from the body.

4. **Olive Leaf (Olea europaea):** Olive leaf extract contains oleuropein, a compound known for its antioxidant and anti-inflammatory properties. Research suggests that olive leaf extract may help lower blood pressure by improving endothelial function and reducing arterial stiffness.

5. **Celery Seed (Apium graveolens):** Celery seed extract contains compounds such as phthalides, which have been shown to have antihypertensive effects. Celery seed may help relax smooth muscle tissue in the blood vessels, leading to improved blood flow and lower blood pressure.

Mechanisms of Action:

The mechanisms by which herbs support blood pressure regulation are diverse and multifaceted. Some of the key mechanisms include:

- **Vasodilation:** Many herbs exert their antihypertensive effects by promoting the relaxation and dilation of blood vessels, thereby reducing peripheral resistance and lowering blood pressure.

- **Diuretic Action:** Certain herbs have diuretic properties, which help increase urine production and promote the excretion of excess fluid and sodium from the body, leading to a decrease in blood volume and blood pressure.

- **Antioxidant Activity:** Antioxidant compounds found in herbs help protect blood vessels from oxidative damage and inflammation, which can contribute to hypertension and cardiovascular disease.

- **Stress Reduction:** Adaptogenic herbs help the body adapt to stress and promote relaxation, which can indirectly lower blood pressure by reducing stress hormone levels and promoting overall cardiovascular health.

Integration into a Holistic Approach:

Dr. Barbara emphasizes the importance of integrating herbal remedies into a holistic approach to managing hypertension. This involves addressing not only the physical symptoms but also the underlying causes and contributing factors, including lifestyle habits, stress, diet, and emotional well-being. Herbal remedies can complement other holistic modalities such as nutrition, exercise, mindfulness practices, and stress management techniques to support overall cardiovascular health.

Conclusion:

The healing power of herbs offers a natural and holistic approach to supporting blood pressure regulation and cardiovascular health. By leveraging the therapeutic properties of herbs such as hawthorn, garlic, hibiscus, olive leaf, and celery seed, individuals can take proactive steps to manage hypertension and promote overall well-being. When used as part of a comprehensive holistic approach, herbal remedies can provide gentle yet effective support for maintaining healthy blood pressure levels and reducing the risk of cardiovascular disease.

CHAPTER FOUR

Preparing for Your Healing Journey: Setting Goals and Gathering Herbal Ingredients

Embarking on a healing journey to manage high blood pressure through herbal remedies requires careful planning and preparation. Dr. Barbara emphasizes the importance of setting clear goals and gathering the necessary herbal ingredients to support your journey to wellness. In this guide, we'll explore the process of goal setting, selecting appropriate herbs, and ensuring you have the essential ingredients to begin your healing journey effectively.

Setting Clear Goals:

Before starting any healing regimen, it's essential to establish clear and achievable goals. Consider what you hope to accomplish through herbal therapy and how you envision your health and well-being improving. Some common goals for managing high blood pressure with herbs may include:

1. **Lowering Blood Pressure:** Set a target range for your blood pressure readings and aim to achieve and maintain these levels through herbal remedies and lifestyle modifications.

2. **Reducing Medication Dependence:** If you're currently taking medication for hypertension, you may aim to reduce your

reliance on these medications over time by incorporating herbal remedies and adopting a healthier lifestyle.

3. **Improving Overall Cardiovascular Health:** Focus on supporting not just your blood pressure but also your overall cardiovascular health, including reducing inflammation, improving circulation, and supporting heart function.

4. **Enhancing Quality of Life:** Consider how managing your blood pressure naturally with herbs can improve your quality of life, including reducing symptoms such as headaches, fatigue, and dizziness associated with hypertension.

By setting specific, measurable, achievable, relevant, and time-bound (SMART) goals, you can track your progress and stay motivated throughout your healing journey.

Selecting Herbal Ingredients:

Once you've established your goals, it's time to select the herbal ingredients that will support your efforts to manage high blood pressure. Dr. Barbara recommends choosing herbs based on their known therapeutic properties and compatibility with your individual health needs. Some key considerations when selecting herbal ingredients include:

1. **Antihypertensive Properties:** Look for herbs that have been traditionally used to lower blood pressure, such as hawthorn, garlic, hibiscus, olive leaf, and celery seed. These

herbs contain bioactive compounds that help regulate blood pressure levels through various mechanisms, including vasodilation, diuretic action, and antioxidant activity.

2. **Safety and Compatibility:** Ensure that the herbs you select are safe for your individual health profile and compatible with any medications or existing health conditions you may have. Consult with a qualified herbalist or healthcare provider to assess potential herb-drug interactions and contraindications.

3. **Quality and Purity:** Choose high-quality herbal products from reputable sources to ensure potency, purity, and efficacy. Look for organic or wildcrafted herbs that have been responsibly sourced and processed to retain their therapeutic properties.

4. **Formulation and Dosage:** Consider the form in which you prefer to consume herbal remedies, whether as teas, tinctures, capsules, or extracts. Follow recommended dosage guidelines provided by reputable sources or healthcare professionals to ensure safe and effective use.

Gathering Essential Ingredients:

Once you've identified the herbal ingredients you plan to use, gather everything you'll need to begin your healing journey. This may include:

1. **Herbal Supplements:** Purchase or prepare herbal supplements in the appropriate form and dosage for your needs. You may choose to purchase pre-made herbal products from reputable manufacturers or prepare your own herbal teas, tinctures, or capsules at home.

2. **Dried Herbs:** If you prefer to use whole herbs, purchase high-quality dried herbs from reputable suppliers. Store them in a cool, dark place away from moisture to preserve their potency and freshness.

3. **Supplies and Equipment:** Gather any supplies and equipment you'll need to prepare and administer herbal remedies, such as teapots, infusers, measuring spoons, and storage containers.

4. **Educational Resources:** Invest in educational resources such as books, articles, or online courses to deepen your understanding of herbal medicine and empower yourself to make informed decisions about your health.

By setting clear goals, selecting appropriate herbal ingredients, and gathering essential supplies, you'll be well-prepared to embark on your healing journey to manage high blood pressure with herbs. Remember to approach your journey with patience, consistency, and a commitment to holistic wellness, and consult with qualified healthcare professionals as needed along the way. With dedication and perseverance, you can achieve your health goals and experience the transformative power of herbal medicine.

CHAPTER FIVE

Selecting the Right Herbs: Dr. Barbara's Recommended Ingredients for Managing High Blood Pressure

Dr. Barbara, a holistic health practitioner, emphasizes the importance of selecting the right herbs to effectively manage high blood pressure (hypertension). Herbs possess a diverse range of therapeutic properties that can support cardiovascular health and promote blood pressure regulation. In this guide, we'll explore Dr. Barbara's recommended herbal ingredients for managing hypertension and their mechanisms of action.

Hawthorn (Crataegus spp.):

Hawthorn is a well-known herb traditionally used to support heart health and regulate blood pressure. It contains bioactive compounds such as flavonoids and procyanidins, which have vasodilatory effects, helping to relax and dilate blood vessels. This can lead to improved blood flow and reduced blood pressure levels. Hawthorn also has antioxidant properties, protecting the cardiovascular system from oxidative damage and inflammation.

Garlic (Allium sativum):

Garlic is another popular herb with potent cardiovascular benefits, including its ability to lower blood pressure. It contains sulfur compounds such as allicin, which have been shown to have hypotensive effects by promoting vasodilation and reducing peripheral resistance. Garlic supplementation may help lower both systolic and diastolic blood pressure levels, making it a valuable addition to a hypertension management regimen.

Hibiscus (Hibiscus sabdariffa):

Hibiscus tea is rich in antioxidants, including anthocyanins and polyphenols, which have been linked to reductions in blood pressure. Hibiscus may also have diuretic effects, promoting the excretion of excess fluid and sodium from the body, which can help lower blood volume and blood pressure. Consuming hibiscus tea regularly may contribute to overall cardiovascular health and blood pressure regulation.

Olive Leaf (Olea europaea):

Olive leaf extract is gaining recognition for its cardiovascular benefits, including its potential to lower blood pressure. It contains oleuropein, a compound known for its antioxidant and anti-inflammatory properties. Olive leaf extract may help improve endothelial function, reduce arterial stiffness, and lower blood pressure levels. Incorporating olive leaf extract into your herbal regimen can support overall cardiovascular health and hypertension management.

Celery Seed (Apium graveolens):

Celery seed extract contains compounds such as phthalides, which have been shown to have antihypertensive effects. Celery seed may help relax smooth muscle tissue in the blood vessels, leading to improved blood flow and lower blood pressure. Additionally, celery seed has diuretic properties, promoting the excretion of excess fluid and sodium from the body. Including celery seed extract in your herbal protocol can complement other antihypertensive herbs and support blood pressure regulation.

Ginger (Zingiber officinale):

Ginger is a versatile herb with a wide range of health benefits, including its potential to lower blood pressure. It contains bioactive compounds such as gingerols and shogaols, which have been shown to have vasodilatory effects and inhibit platelet aggregation. Ginger may help improve blood circulation, reduce inflammation, and lower blood pressure levels when consumed regularly as part of a balanced diet and herbal regimen.

Choosing the Right Herbs for You:

When selecting herbs for managing high blood pressure, it's essential to consider your individual health needs, preferences, and any potential contraindications. Consult with a qualified herbalist or healthcare provider to determine the most appropriate herbal ingredients and dosage for your unique circumstances. Integrating these recommended herbs into a holistic approach to managing hypertension can support cardiovascular health, promote blood pressure regulation, and contribute to overall well-being.

CHAPTER SIX

Crafting Healing Recipes: Herbal Formulas and Teas Designed to Lower Blood Pressure Naturally

Crafting healing recipes using herbal formulas and teas offers a natural and holistic approach to managing high blood pressure (hypertension). Dr. Barbara, a holistic health practitioner, advocates for the strategic use of herbs to support cardiovascular health and promote blood pressure regulation. In this guide, we'll explore herbal formulas and teas designed to lower blood pressure naturally, incorporating Dr. Barbara's recommendations and insights.

Herbal Formula for Blood Pressure Regulation:

Creating a herbal formula for blood pressure regulation involves combining specific herbs known for their antihypertensive properties. Here's a simple herbal formula to consider:

Ingredients:

- Hawthorn (Crataegus spp.) - 1 part

- Garlic (Allium sativum) - 1 part

- Hibiscus (Hibiscus sabdariffa) - 1 part

- Olive Leaf (Olea europaea) - 1 part

- Celery Seed (Apium graveolens) - 1 part

Instructions:

1. Combine equal parts of dried hawthorn berries and leaves, garlic cloves, hibiscus flowers, olive leaf, and celery seed in a large mixing bowl.

2. Thoroughly mix the herbs together until well combined.

3. Store the herbal formula in an airtight container in a cool, dark place away from moisture.

Usage:

- To prepare a tea, steep 1 teaspoon of the herbal formula in 8 ounces of hot water for 10-15 minutes. Strain and drink the tea 1-2 times daily.

- Alternatively, the herbal formula can be encapsulated for convenient consumption. Consult with a qualified herbalist or healthcare provider for appropriate dosage recommendations.

Herbal Tea for Blood Pressure Regulation:

Herbal teas offer a convenient and enjoyable way to incorporate medicinal herbs into your daily routine. Here's a soothing herbal tea recipe designed to lower blood pressure naturally:

Ingredients:

- 1 teaspoon dried hawthorn berries

- 1 teaspoon dried garlic flakes

- 1 teaspoon dried hibiscus flowers

- 1 teaspoon dried olive leaf

- 1 teaspoon dried celery seed

- 2 cups filtered water

Instructions:

1. In a small saucepan, bring the filtered water to a gentle boil.

2. Add the dried hawthorn berries, garlic flakes, hibiscus flowers, olive leaf, and celery seed to the boiling water.

3. Reduce the heat to low and simmer the herbs for 10-15 minutes, allowing the flavors to infuse.

4. Remove the saucepan from the heat and let the herbal tea steep for an additional 5 minutes.

5. Strain the tea into a teapot or serving pitcher, discarding the spent herbs.

6. Serve the herbal tea hot or chilled, according to your preference.

Usage:

- Enjoy 1-2 cups of the herbal tea daily as part of your hypertension management regimen.

- Adjust the strength and flavor of the tea by increasing or decreasing the amount of herbs used and the steeping time.

Tips for Crafting Healing Recipes:

1. **Quality Ingredients:** Use high-quality, organic herbs sourced from reputable suppliers to ensure potency and efficacy.

2. **Dosage Considerations:** Consult with a qualified herbalist or healthcare provider to determine appropriate dosages based on your individual health needs and goals.

3. **Consistency:** Incorporate herbal formulas and teas into your daily routine consistently to maximize their therapeutic benefits.

4. **Monitor Progress:** Keep track of your blood pressure readings and overall health to assess the effectiveness of the herbal remedies and make any necessary adjustments.

By crafting healing recipes using herbal formulas and teas specifically designed to lower blood pressure naturally, you can take proactive steps to support cardiovascular health and promote overall well-being. Experiment with different combinations of herbs and enjoy the transformative power of herbal medicine on your healing journey.

CHAPTER SEVEN

Incorporating Additional Lifestyle Changes: Enhancing the Effectiveness of Herbal Treatment

While herbal treatments can play a significant role in managing high blood pressure (hypertension), incorporating additional lifestyle changes can further enhance their effectiveness and promote overall cardiovascular health. Dr. Barbara, a holistic health practitioner, advocates for a comprehensive approach that integrates herbal remedies with lifestyle modifications to optimize blood pressure regulation. In this guide, we'll explore key lifestyle changes that can complement herbal treatment and contribute to long-term hypertension management.

1. Adopting a Healthy Diet:

A balanced and nutritious diet is essential for maintaining optimal blood pressure levels and supporting overall cardiovascular health. Dr. Barbara recommends the following dietary guidelines:

- **Emphasize Plant-Based Foods:** Fill your plate with fruits, vegetables, whole grains, legumes, nuts, and seeds, which are rich in vitamins, minerals, fiber, and antioxidants.

- **Limit Sodium Intake:** Reduce your consumption of high-sodium foods such as processed foods, canned soups, and salty snacks, as excessive sodium intake can contribute to hypertension.

- **Moderate Alcohol Consumption:** Limit alcohol consumption to moderate levels, as excessive alcohol intake can raise blood pressure and increase the risk of cardiovascular disease.

- **Monitor Potassium and Magnesium Intake:** Incorporate potassium-rich foods like bananas, leafy greens, and sweet potatoes, as well as magnesium-rich foods like nuts, seeds, and whole grains, which can help lower blood pressure.

2. Engaging in Regular Physical Activity:

Regular exercise is an integral component of hypertension management, as it helps strengthen the heart, improve circulation, and lower blood pressure. Dr. Barbara recommends the following exercise guidelines:

- **Aim for at Least 150 Minutes of Moderate-Intensity Exercise Weekly:** Engage in activities such as brisk walking, cycling, swimming, or dancing to promote cardiovascular fitness and blood pressure control.

- **Incorporate Strength Training:** Include strength training exercises at least twice a week to build muscle mass, improve metabolism, and enhance overall physical function.

- **Stay Active Throughout the Day:** Incorporate movement into your daily routine by taking short walks, using stairs instead of elevators, and participating in active hobbies or household chores.

3. Managing Stress and Prioritizing Relaxation:

Chronic stress can contribute to hypertension by increasing heart rate, constricting blood vessels, and raising blood pressure. Dr. Barbara recommends the following stress management techniques:

- **Practice Mindfulness Meditation:** Engage in mindfulness meditation, deep breathing exercises, or progressive muscle relaxation to promote relaxation and reduce stress levels.

- **Prioritize Sleep:** Aim for 7-9 hours of quality sleep per night to support overall health and well-being. Establish a consistent sleep schedule, create a relaxing bedtime routine, and create a conducive sleep environment.

- **Engage in Stress-Relieving Activities:** Participate in activities that bring you joy and relaxation, such as spending time in nature, practicing yoga or tai chi, listening to music, or spending time with loved ones.

4. Maintaining a Healthy Weight:

Maintaining a healthy weight is important for blood pressure management and overall cardiovascular health. Dr. Barbara recommends the following strategies for weight management:

- **Focus on Sustainable Weight Loss:** Aim for gradual, sustainable weight loss through a combination of dietary changes, regular exercise, and lifestyle modifications.

- **Monitor Portion Sizes:** Pay attention to portion sizes and practice mindful eating to avoid overeating and promote satiety.

- **Seek Support:** Consider working with a registered dietitian, nutritionist, or weight loss coach to develop a personalized plan tailored to your individual needs and goals.

5. Avoiding Tobacco and Limiting Caffeine Intake:

Tobacco use and excessive caffeine intake can contribute to hypertension and cardiovascular disease. Dr. Barbara recommends the following strategies for tobacco and caffeine management:

- **Quit Smoking:** If you smoke, seek support to quit smoking and improve your cardiovascular health. Consider nicotine replacement therapy, counseling, or support groups to aid in smoking cessation.

- **Limit Caffeine Consumption:** Reduce your intake of caffeinated beverages such as coffee, tea, and energy drinks, as excessive caffeine consumption can elevate blood pressure and contribute to cardiovascular problems.

Conclusion:

Incorporating additional lifestyle changes alongside herbal treatment can significantly enhance the effectiveness of hypertension management and promote overall cardiovascular health. By adopting a healthy diet, engaging in regular physical activity, managing stress, maintaining a healthy weight, and avoiding tobacco and excessive caffeine intake, you can synergistically support the therapeutic effects of herbal remedies and achieve optimal blood pressure control. Dr. Barbara's holistic approach emphasizes the importance of addressing the root causes of hypertension and empowering individuals to take proactive steps toward long-term wellness and vitality.

CHAPTER EIGHT

Navigating Challenges: Tips for Adjusting to Herbal Remedies and Monitoring Blood Pressure Levels

Embarking on a journey to manage high blood pressure (hypertension) with herbal remedies can bring about positive changes in your health and well-being. However, navigating this path may also present challenges as you adjust to new routines and monitor your blood pressure levels. Dr. Barbara, a holistic health practitioner, offers valuable tips for overcoming these challenges and optimizing your hypertension management journey. In this guide, we'll explore strategies for adjusting to herbal remedies and effectively monitoring your blood pressure levels.

1. Start Slowly and Gradually:

When incorporating herbal remedies into your routine, start with small doses and gradually increase them over time. This allows your body to adjust to the herbs and reduces the risk of potential side effects. Pay attention to how your body responds and make adjustments as needed under the guidance of a qualified herbalist or healthcare provider.

2. Stay Consistent:

Consistency is key when using herbal remedies for hypertension management. Take your herbal supplements or teas regularly as directed to maintain steady blood pressure control. Set reminders or incorporate them into your daily routine to ensure you don't miss doses. Consistent use over time can yield the most significant benefits for your cardiovascular health.

3. Listen to Your Body:

Pay attention to how your body responds to herbal remedies and monitor for any signs of discomfort or adverse reactions. If you experience any unusual symptoms, such as headaches, nausea, or dizziness, consult with a healthcare professional promptly. It's essential to address any concerns and make adjustments to your herbal regimen as needed to ensure your safety and well-being.

4. Monitor Blood Pressure Levels:

Regular monitoring of your blood pressure levels is crucial for tracking your progress and assessing the effectiveness of herbal treatment. Invest in a reliable blood pressure monitor for home use and follow these tips for accurate readings:

- **Consistent Timing:** Take your blood pressure readings at the same time each day, preferably in the morning before consuming any food or beverages.

- **Relaxation:** Sit quietly for at least 5 minutes before taking your blood pressure measurement to ensure accuracy. Avoid talking or engaging in any strenuous activities during this time.

- **Proper Technique:** Position yourself comfortably with your back supported, feet flat on the floor, and arm supported at heart level. Follow the instructions provided with your blood pressure monitor for correct usage.

- **Record Keeping:** Keep a log of your blood pressure readings, along with any relevant information such as herbal doses, dietary changes, exercise habits, and stress levels. This record can help you and your healthcare provider track trends and make informed decisions about your hypertension management plan.

5. Stay Informed and Seek Support:

Educate yourself about herbal remedies, hypertension management, and lifestyle modifications to empower yourself on your healing journey. Stay informed about potential herb-drug interactions and contraindications, and don't hesitate to ask questions or seek guidance from qualified herbalists or healthcare providers. Joining support groups or online communities can also provide valuable resources and encouragement from others on similar journeys.

Conclusion:

Navigating the challenges of adjusting to herbal remedies and monitoring blood pressure levels requires patience, diligence, and self-awareness. By starting slowly, staying consistent, listening to your body, monitoring blood pressure levels, staying informed, and seeking support when needed, you can overcome obstacles and achieve optimal results in managing hypertension naturally with herbs. Dr. Barbara's holistic approach emphasizes the importance of personalized care, empowerment, and collaboration in achieving long-term cardiovascular health and well-being.

CHAPTER NINE

Success Stories: Real-Life Accounts of Individuals Who Have Improved Their High Blood Pressure Through Herbal Treatment

Real-life success stories provide valuable inspiration and motivation for individuals seeking to manage high blood pressure (hypertension) through herbal treatment. Dr. Barbara, a holistic health practitioner, shares stories of individuals who have experienced significant improvements in their blood pressure levels and overall health by incorporating herbal remedies into their daily routines. These success stories highlight the transformative power of herbal medicine and the potential for positive outcomes in hypertension management. Let's explore some real-life accounts of individuals who have successfully improved their high blood pressure through herbal treatment:

Case Study 1: Sarah's Journey to Blood Pressure Control

Sarah, a 52-year-old woman, had struggled with high blood pressure for several years despite taking multiple medications. Concerned about the side effects and limited effectiveness of conventional treatments, she decided to explore alternative approaches. With guidance from Dr. Barbara, Sarah began incorporating herbal remedies into her daily routine.

Sarah started drinking a hibiscus tea blend recommended by Dr. Barbara, which she found enjoyable and easy to incorporate into her morning routine. She also started taking a garlic supplement and using olive leaf extract regularly. Alongside herbal treatment, Sarah made significant lifestyle changes, including adopting a healthier diet, engaging in regular exercise, and practicing stress-reduction techniques.

Over time, Sarah noticed gradual improvements in her blood pressure readings. Her systolic and diastolic blood pressure levels began to decrease steadily, and she experienced fewer fluctuations throughout the day. Encouraged by her progress, Sarah continued to follow her herbal regimen and lifestyle modifications.

After several months of consistent effort, Sarah's blood pressure readings had stabilized within the normal range, and she was able to reduce her reliance on medication with the approval of her healthcare provider. She reported feeling more energetic, focused, and empowered to take control of her health naturally.

Case Study 2: John's Herbal Healing Journey

John, a 65-year-old man, had been diagnosed with hypertension and struggled to find an effective treatment regimen that suited his needs. Dissatisfied with the side effects of prescription medications, he sought alternative solutions and found Dr. Barbara's holistic approach to hypertension management.

Under Dr. Barbara's guidance, John began incorporating a customized herbal formula into his daily routine, which included hawthorn, garlic, celery seed, and olive leaf. He also started drinking a hibiscus tea blend and made dietary changes to reduce his sodium intake and increase his consumption of potassium-rich foods.

As John continued to follow his herbal regimen and lifestyle modifications, he noticed gradual improvements in his blood pressure readings. His hypertension became more manageable, and he experienced fewer symptoms such as headaches and fatigue. John's healthcare provider was impressed by his progress and gradually adjusted his medication dosage accordingly.

With dedication and perseverance, John was able to achieve significant improvements in his blood pressure levels and overall cardiovascular health. He attributed his success to the holistic approach advocated by Dr. Barbara, which addressed the root causes of his hypertension and empowered him to take an active role in his healing journey.

Conclusion:

These real-life success stories demonstrate the transformative potential of herbal treatment in managing high blood pressure naturally. By incorporating herbal remedies into their daily routines and making lifestyle modifications, individuals like Sarah and John were able to achieve significant improvements in their blood pressure levels and overall well-being. Their journeys highlight the importance of personalized care, consistency, and empowerment in achieving positive outcomes in hypertension management. Dr. Barbara's holistic approach offers hope and inspiration to those seeking natural solutions for hypertension and encourages them to embark on their own healing journeys with confidence and optimism.

CHAPTER TEN

Beyond Herbal Remedies: Integrating Dr. Barbara's Principles for Long-Term Blood Pressure Management and Overall Health

Dr. Barbara's holistic approach to managing high blood pressure (hypertension) extends beyond herbal remedies to encompass a comprehensive framework for long-term health and wellness. By integrating Dr. Barbara's principles into your daily life, you can optimize blood pressure management, promote cardiovascular health, and enhance overall well-being. Let's explore key principles for long-term blood pressure management and holistic health based on Dr. Barbara's teachings:

1. Holistic Lifestyle Modification:

Dr. Barbara emphasizes the importance of adopting a holistic lifestyle that addresses the physical, emotional, mental, and spiritual aspects of health. This includes:

- **Nutrition:** Focus on a balanced diet rich in fruits, vegetables, whole grains, lean proteins, and healthy fats. Limit processed foods, refined sugars, and excessive sodium intake. Pay attention to portion sizes and mindful eating habits.

- **Physical Activity:** Engage in regular exercise to promote cardiovascular fitness, strengthen the heart, and improve blood circulation. Aim for a combination of aerobic exercise, strength training, and flexibility exercises tailored to your fitness level and preferences.

- **Stress Management:** Practice stress-reduction techniques such as mindfulness meditation, deep breathing exercises, yoga, tai chi, or progressive muscle relaxation. Prioritize self-care activities, hobbies, and leisure pursuits that bring joy and relaxation.

- **Quality Sleep:** Prioritize sleep hygiene and establish a consistent sleep schedule to ensure adequate rest and recovery. Create a calming bedtime routine, minimize exposure to screens before bed, and create a conducive sleep environment.

2. Mind-Body Connection:

Dr. Barbara recognizes the interconnectedness of the mind and body and the profound impact of thoughts, emotions, and beliefs on health. Cultivate a positive mindset and emotional resilience through practices such as:

- **Mindfulness:** Cultivate present-moment awareness and non-judgmental acceptance of thoughts, feelings, and sensations. Practice mindfulness meditation, mindful eating, and mindful movement to enhance self-awareness and reduce stress.

- **Emotional Well-being:** Nurture supportive relationships, express gratitude, and engage in activities that bring joy, fulfillment, and a sense of purpose. Seek professional support or counseling if needed to address underlying emotional issues or trauma.

3. Environmental Awareness:

Dr. Barbara emphasizes the importance of creating a healthy and supportive environment that promotes well-being and vitality. Consider the following factors:

- **Toxic Exposure:** Minimize exposure to environmental toxins such as air pollution, household chemicals, pesticides, and electromagnetic radiation. Choose natural and eco-friendly products whenever possible and support sustainable practices.

- **Nature Connection:** Spend time in nature regularly to recharge, reduce stress, and promote overall well-being. Take walks in parks, forests, or beaches, practice outdoor activities, and cultivate a deeper connection with the natural world.

4. Self-Empowerment and Education:

Dr. Barbara empowers individuals to take an active role in their health and well-being by providing education, resources, and support. Take ownership of your health journey by:

- **Self-Education:** Stay informed about holistic health principles, nutrition, herbal medicine, and lifestyle interventions. Seek reliable sources of information, attend workshops or seminars, and continue learning to deepen your understanding.

- **Self-Advocacy:** Advocate for your health needs and preferences in collaboration with healthcare providers. Ask questions, express concerns, and actively participate in decision-making regarding your treatment plan and wellness goals.

5. Cultivating Resilience and Adaptability:

Dr. Barbara encourages individuals to embrace change, adapt to challenges, and cultivate resilience in the face of adversity. Develop coping strategies and resilience-building practices such as:

- **Flexibility:** Embrace flexibility and adaptability in your daily routines, goals, and expectations. Be open to new experiences, perspectives, and opportunities for growth.

- **Optimism:** Cultivate a positive outlook and maintain optimism in the face of setbacks or obstacles. Focus on solutions, strengths, and possibilities rather than dwelling on problems or limitations.

BONUS: SOME HERBAL REMEDIES TO KNOW

Bladderwrack:

Definition: Bladderwrack is a type of seaweed or marine algae commonly used in traditional medicine and as a dietary supplement. It's known for its potential health benefits, particularly related to thyroid health and weight management.

Ingredients: Bladderwrack contains various nutrients, including iodine, vitamins, minerals, and antioxidants. The primary active components are iodine and fucoidan, a type of carbohydrate found in brown seaweeds.

How to Prepare: Bladderwrack supplements are available in various forms, including capsules, powders, and liquid extracts. They can be taken orally with water or added to smoothies and other beverages.

Dosage: The appropriate dosage of bladderwrack can vary based on factors such as age, health status, and the specific product being used. It's essential to follow the recommended dosage on the product label or consult with a healthcare professional for personalized guidance.

How to Use: Bladderwrack supplements are typically taken orally, either with water or mixed into food or beverages. It's important to follow the instructions on the product label and avoid exceeding the recommended dosage.

Side Effects: While bladderwrack is generally considered safe for most people when used in moderation, excessive intake of iodine from bladderwrack supplements can cause thyroid dysfunction and other adverse effects. Individuals with thyroid disorders, iodine sensitivity, or certain medical conditions should exercise caution and consult with a healthcare provider before using bladderwrack supplements. Common side effects may include digestive upset, allergic reactions, or interactions with medications.

Blood Purifier:

Definition: Blood purifiers are herbal remedies or dietary supplements believed to cleanse or detoxify the blood, often promoting overall health and well-being. They are thought to support the body's natural detoxification processes and improve blood circulation.

Ingredients: Blood purifiers may contain a variety of herbs and botanical extracts known for their purported cleansing and detoxifying properties. Common ingredients include burdock root, red clover, dandelion root, and yellow dock root, among others.

How to Prepare: Blood purifiers are typically available in various forms, including capsules, tablets, powders, and liquid extracts. They are usually taken orally with water or juice, following the recommended dosage on the product label.

Dosage: The dosage of blood purifiers can vary depending on the specific product and individual needs. It's important to adhere to the recommended dosage on the product label or consult with a healthcare professional for personalized guidance.

How to Use: Blood purifiers are typically taken orally, either with water or mixed into beverages. They are often used as part of a detoxification regimen or to support overall health and vitality.

Side Effects: While blood purifiers are generally considered safe for most people when used as directed, some individuals may experience side effects such as digestive discomfort, allergic reactions, or interactions with medications. It's important to consult with a healthcare provider before starting any new supplement regimen, especially if you have underlying health conditions or are taking medications.

Blue Vervain:

Definition: Blue vervain, also known as Verbena hastata, is a perennial herb native to North America. It has been used in traditional medicine for centuries to treat various ailments, including anxiety, insomnia, and digestive issues.

Ingredients: Blue vervain contains several active compounds, including aucubin, verbenalin, and volatile oils. These compounds are believed to contribute to the herb's medicinal properties.

How to Prepare: Blue vervain is typically consumed as a tea or tincture. To make tea, dried blue vervain leaves and flowers are steeped in hot water for several minutes before being strained and consumed. Tinctures are prepared by steeping the herb in alcohol or vinegar to extract its active compounds.

Dosage: The appropriate dosage of blue vervain can vary depending on factors such as age, health status, and the specific preparation being used. It's important to follow the recommended dosage on the product label or consult with a qualified herbalist or healthcare professional for personalized guidance.

How to Use: Blue vervain tea or tincture is typically taken orally. It can be consumed on its own or mixed with honey or other herbal teas for added flavor.

Side Effects: While blue vervain is generally considered safe for most people when used in moderation, excessive intake may cause digestive upset or allergic reactions in some individuals. Pregnant or breastfeeding women should avoid blue vervain due to its potential to stimulate uterine contractions. As with any herbal remedy, it's important to consult with a healthcare provider before using blue vervain, especially if you have underlying health conditions or are taking medications.

Bromide Plus Powder:

Definition: Bromide Plus Powder is a dietary supplement formulated to support thyroid health and promote overall well-being. It typically contains a blend of herbs and minerals that are believed to have beneficial effects on thyroid function.

Ingredients: Bromide Plus Powder often contains a combination of herbs such as bladderwrack, sea moss, and burdock root, along with minerals like iodine and potassium phosphate. These ingredients are thought to support thyroid function and maintain optimal iodine levels in the body.

How to Prepare: Bromide Plus Powder is usually mixed with water or juice to create a drinkable solution. It's important to follow the instructions on the product label for dosage and preparation.

Dosage: The dosage of Bromide Plus Powder can vary depending on the specific product and individual needs. It's crucial to consult with a healthcare professional or follow the recommended dosage on the product label to avoid potential side effects.

How to Use: Bromide Plus Powder is typically taken orally by mixing the recommended dosage with water or juice. It's important to shake or stir the mixture well before consuming it to ensure even distribution of the ingredients.

Side Effects: While Bromide Plus Powder is generally considered safe when used as directed, some individuals may experience side effects such as digestive discomfort or allergic reactions to certain ingredients. It's essential to consult with a healthcare provider before starting any new supplement regimen, especially if you have underlying health conditions or are taking medications.

Bugleweed:

Definition: Bugleweed, also known as Lycopusvirginicus, is a perennial herb native to North America and Europe. It has been used in traditional medicine to treat various conditions, including hyperthyroidism, anxiety, and insomnia.

Ingredients: Bugleweed contains several active compounds, including lithospermic acid, phenolic acids, and flavonoids. These compounds are believed to contribute to the herb's medicinal properties, particularly its ability to regulate thyroid function.

How to Prepare: Bugleweed is commonly consumed as a tea or tincture. To make tea, dried bugleweed leaves and flowers are steeped in hot water for several minutes before being strained and consumed. Tinctures are prepared by steeping the herb in alcohol or vinegar to extract its active compounds.

Dosage: The appropriate dosage of bugleweed can vary depending on factors such as age, health status, and the specific preparation being used. It's important to follow the recommended dosage on the product label or consult with a qualified herbalist or healthcare professional for personalized guidance.

How to Use: Bugleweed tea or tincture is typically taken orally. It can be consumed on its own or mixed with honey or other herbal teas for added flavor.

Side Effects: While bugleweed is generally considered safe for most people when used in moderation, excessive intake may cause digestive upset or allergic reactions in some individuals. Pregnant or breastfeeding women should avoid bugleweed due to its potential to stimulate uterine contractions. As with any herbal remedy, it's important to consult with a healthcare provider before using bugleweed, especially if you have underlying health conditions or are taking medications.

Cocolmeca:

Definition: Cocolmeca, also known as Smilax ornata or sarsaparilla, is a flowering vine native to Mexico and Central America. It has been used traditionally in Mexican and Central American folk medicine for its purported medicinal properties.

Ingredients: Cocolmeca contains various bioactive compounds, including saponins, flavonoids, and plant sterols. These compounds are believed to contribute to the herb's medicinal properties, including its potential as a diuretic, blood purifier, and anti-inflammatory agent.

How to Prepare: Cocolmeca is commonly prepared and consumed as an herbal tea or decoction. To make tea, dried cocolmeca roots or leaves are steeped in hot water for several minutes before being strained and consumed. Decoctions involve boiling the roots or leaves in water to extract their active compounds.

Dosage: The appropriate dosage of cocolmeca can vary depending on factors such as age, health status, and the specific preparation being used. It's important to follow the recommended dosage on the product label or consult with a qualified herbalist or healthcare professional for personalized guidance.

How to Use: Cocolmeca tea or decoction is typically taken orally. It can also be used topically for certain skin conditions. It's important to use cocolmeca products as directed and to discontinue use if any adverse effects occur.

Side Effects: Cocolmeca is generally considered safe for most people when used in moderate amounts. However, excessive intake may lead to digestive upset or other adverse effects. It may also interact with certain medications or have adverse effects in individuals with certain health conditions. It's important to use cocolmeca under the guidance of a healthcare professional and to discontinue use if any adverse effects occur.

Contribo:

Definition: Contribo, also known as Aristolochiatrilobata, is a vine native to the Caribbean and Central America. It has been used traditionally in folk medicine for various purposes, including as a remedy for digestive issues, inflammation, and pain relief.

Ingredients: Contribo contains several bioactive compounds, including aristolochic acids, flavonoids, and alkaloids. These compounds are believed to contribute to the herb's medicinal properties, including its potential as an anti-inflammatory and analgesic agent.

How to Prepare: Contribo is typically prepared and consumed as an herbal tea or decoction. To make tea, dried contribo leaves or stems are steeped in hot water for several minutes before being strained and consumed. Decoctions involve boiling the leaves or stems in water to extract their active compounds.

Dosage: The appropriate dosage of contribo can vary depending on factors such as age, health status, and the specific preparation being used. It's important to follow the recommended dosage on the product label or consult with a qualified herbalist or healthcare professional for personalized guidance.

How to Use: Contribo tea or decoction is typically taken orally. It's important to use contribo products as directed and to discontinue use if any adverse effects occur.

Side Effects: Contribo contains aristolochic acids, which have been associated with serious adverse effects, including kidney damage and cancer. Due to these safety concerns, the use of contribo is highly discouraged, and it's important to avoid products containing aristolochic acids. Individuals should seek alternative remedies for their health needs.

Dandelion Root:

Definition: Dandelion, scientifically known as Taraxacum officinale, is a common flowering plant found worldwide. While often considered a pesky weed, dandelion has a long history of use in traditional medicine for its various health benefits.

Ingredients: Dandelion root contains several bioactive compounds, including sesquiterpene lactones, triterpenes, flavonoids, and polysaccharides. These compounds are believed to contribute to the herb's medicinal properties, including its potential as a diuretic, digestive aid, and liver tonic.

How to Prepare: Dandelion root can be prepared and consumed in various forms, including teas, tinctures, capsules, and extracts. To make tea, dried dandelion root is steeped in hot water for several minutes before being strained and consumed. Tinctures are prepared by steeping the root in alcohol or vinegar to extract its active compounds.

Dosage: The appropriate dosage of dandelion root can vary depending on factors such as age, health status, and the specific preparation being used. It's important to follow the recommended dosage on the product label or consult with a qualified herbalist or healthcare professional for personalized guidance.

How to Use: Dandelion root tea, tincture, or capsules are typically taken orally. It's important to use dandelion root products as directed and to discontinue use if any adverse effects occur.

Side Effects: Dandelion root is generally considered safe for most people when used in moderate amounts. However, some individuals may experience allergic reactions or digestive upset. It may also interact with certain medications or have adverse effects in individuals with certain health conditions. It's important to use dandelion root under the guidance of a healthcare professional and to discontinue use if any adverse effects occur.

Green Food Plus:

Definition: Green Food Plus is a dietary supplement formulated to provide a concentrated source of nutrients derived from various green plants. It's designed to support overall health and well-being by delivering essential vitamins, minerals, antioxidants, and phytonutrients.

Ingredients: Green Food Plus typically contains a blend of powdered green vegetables, grasses, algae, and other plant-based ingredients. Common ingredients may include wheatgrass, barley grass, spirulina, chlorella, alfalfa, kale, spinach, and broccoli, among others.

How to Prepare: Green Food Plus is usually available in powder form and can be mixed with water, juice, or smoothies. It's important to follow the recommended dosage on the product label and to consume it as part of a balanced diet.

Dosage: The appropriate dosage of Green Food Plus can vary depending on the specific product and individual needs. It's important to follow the recommended dosage on the product label or consult with a healthcare professional for personalized guidance.

How to Use: Green Food Plus powder is typically mixed with water, juice, or smoothies and consumed orally. It's often taken once or twice daily, preferably with meals, to maximize nutrient absorption.

Side Effects: Green Food Plus is generally considered safe for most people when used as directed. However, some individuals may experience digestive upset or allergic reactions to certain ingredients. It's important to consult with a healthcare provider before starting any new supplement regimen, especially if you have underlying health conditions or are taking medications.

Guaco:

Definition: Guaco, also known as Mikania cordata or Mikania glomerata, is a medicinal plant native to Central and South America. It has a long history of use in traditional medicine for its potential therapeutic properties.

Ingredients: Guaco contains several bioactive compounds, including coumarins, flavonoids, tannins, and saponins. These compounds are believed to contribute to the herb's medicinal properties, including its potential as an expectorant, anti-inflammatory, and antispasmodic agent.

How to Prepare: Guaco is typically prepared and consumed as an herbal tea or infusion. To make tea, dried guaco leaves are steeped in hot water for several minutes before being strained and consumed.

Dosage: The appropriate dosage of guaco can vary depending on factors such as age, health status, and the specific preparation being used. It's important to follow the recommended dosage on the product label or consult with a qualified herbalist or healthcare professional for personalized guidance.

How to Use: Guaco tea is typically taken orally. It can be consumed on its own or mixed with honey or other herbal teas for added flavor.

Side Effects: Guaco is generally considered safe for most people when used in moderate amounts. However, some individuals may experience allergic reactions or digestive upset. It may also interact with certain medications or have adverse effects in individuals with certain health conditions. It's important to use guaco under the guidance of a healthcare professional and to discontinue use if any adverse effects occur.

Herban Iron:

Definition: Herban Iron is a dietary supplement designed to provide an easily absorbable form of iron to support healthy iron levels in the body. It's particularly beneficial for individuals with iron deficiency or anemia.

Ingredients: Herban Iron typically contains iron in the form of ferrous bisglycinate, which is a highly bioavailable and gentle form of iron that is less likely to cause digestive upset or constipation compared to other forms of iron. It may also contain other ingredients such as vitamin C to enhance iron absorption.

How to Prepare: Herban Iron is usually available in capsule or liquid form. Capsules are taken orally with water, while liquid forms may be mixed with water or juice before consumption. It's important to follow the recommended dosage on the product label.

Dosage: The appropriate dosage of Herban Iron depends on factors such as age, gender, and the severity of iron deficiency. It's important to consult with a healthcare professional to determine the correct dosage for individual needs.

How to Use: Herban Iron capsules are typically taken orally with water, while liquid forms may be mixed with water or juice before consumption. It's important to take Herban Iron as directed and to avoid taking it with dairy products, antacids, or other substances that may interfere with iron absorption.

Side Effects: While Herban Iron is generally considered safe for most people when used as directed, some individuals may experience mild side effects such as gastrointestinal discomfort or constipation. It's important to consult with a healthcare professional before starting any new supplement regimen, especially if you have underlying health conditions or are taking medications.

Hydrangea:

Definition: Hydrangea, scientifically known as Hydrangea arborescens, is a flowering shrub native to North America. It has been used traditionally in herbal medicine for its potential diuretic and anti-inflammatory properties.

Ingredients: Hydrangea contains several bioactive compounds, including saponins, flavonoids, and glycosides. These compounds are believed to contribute to the herb's medicinal properties, including its potential as a diuretic, kidney tonic, and anti-inflammatory agent.

How to Prepare: Hydrangea root is typically prepared and consumed as an herbal tea or tincture. To make tea, dried hydrangea root is steeped in hot water for several minutes before being strained and consumed. Tinctures are prepared by steeping the root in alcohol or vinegar to extract its active compounds.

Dosage: The appropriate dosage of hydrangea can vary depending on factors such as age, health status, and the specific preparation being used. It's important to follow the recommended dosage on the product label or consult with a qualified herbalist or healthcare professional for personalized guidance.

How to Use: Hydrangea tea or tincture is typically taken orally. It's important to use hydrangea products as directed and to discontinue use if any adverse effects occur.

Side Effects: Hydrangea is generally considered safe for most people when used in moderate amounts. However, some individuals may experience digestive upset or allergic reactions. It may also interact with certain medications or have adverse effects in individuals with certain health conditions. It's important to use hydrangea under the guidance of a healthcare professional and to discontinue use if any adverse effects occur.

Irish Moss:

Definition: Irish Moss, scientifically known as Chondrus crispus, is a species of red algae or seaweed native to the Atlantic coastlines of Europe and North America. It has been used for centuries in traditional Irish and Scottish cuisine, as well as in herbal medicine.

Ingredients: Irish Moss is rich in various nutrients, including iodine, sulfur compounds, vitamins (such as vitamin A, vitamin K, and vitamin B12), minerals (including calcium, magnesium, potassium, and sodium), and polysaccharides (such as carrageenan). These nutrients are believed to contribute to the herb's potential health benefits.

How to Prepare: Irish Moss is typically prepared by soaking it in water to rehydrate and soften it before use. It can be added to soups, stews, smoothies, desserts, and other dishes as a thickening agent or nutritional supplement.

Dosage: The appropriate dosage of Irish Moss can vary depending on factors such as age, health status, and the specific preparation being used. It's important to follow recipes or guidelines for culinary use and to consult with a healthcare professional for guidance on using Irish Moss as a dietary supplement.

How to Use: Irish Moss can be used in culinary applications to add thickness and nutritional value to dishes. It can also be consumed as a dietary supplement in the form of capsules, powders, or extracts.

Side Effects: Irish Moss is generally considered safe for most people when consumed in moderate amounts as part of a balanced diet. However, some individuals may be allergic to seaweed or carrageenan, a compound found in Irish Moss that is used as a food additive. It's important to discontinue use if any adverse effects occur and to consult with a healthcare professional if you have any concerns.

Irish Sea Moss:

Definition: Irish Sea Moss is a term often used interchangeably with Irish Moss, referring to the same species of red algae, Chondrus crispus. It's harvested from the rocky shores of the Atlantic coastlines of Europe and North America.

Ingredients: Irish Sea Moss shares the same nutritional profile as Irish Moss, containing iodine, vitamins, minerals, and polysaccharides. It's valued for its potential health benefits, including supporting thyroid function, boosting immune health, and promoting digestion.

How to Prepare: Irish Sea Moss is prepared in the same way as Irish Moss, by soaking it in water to rehydrate and soften it before use. It can be used in culinary applications or consumed as a dietary supplement.

Dosage: The dosage of Irish Sea Moss depends on the form and intended use. As a dietary supplement, it's important to follow the recommended dosage on the product label or consult with a healthcare professional for personalized guidance.

How to Use: Irish Sea Moss can be used in various culinary applications, including soups, smoothies, desserts, and sauces. It can also be consumed as a dietary supplement in the form of capsules, powders, or extracts.

Side Effects: Similar to Irish Moss, Irish Sea Moss is generally considered safe for most people when consumed in moderate amounts. However, individuals with seaweed allergies or sensitivities to carrageenan should exercise caution. It's important to discontinue use if any adverse effects occur and to consult with a healthcare professional if you have any concerns.

Lymphalin:

Definition: Lymphalin is a herbal supplement formulated to support lymphatic system health. The lymphatic system plays a crucial role in immune function and waste removal in the body, and Lymphalin is designed to promote its proper function.

Ingredients: Lymphalin typically contains a blend of herbs and botanical extracts known for their traditional use in supporting lymphatic system health. Common ingredients may include cleavers, red clover, echinacea, burdock root, and calendula, among others.

How to Prepare: Lymphalin is usually available in capsule or liquid form. Capsules are taken orally with water, while liquid forms may be mixed with water or juice before consumption. It's important to follow the recommended dosage on the product label.

Dosage: The appropriate dosage of Lymphalin can vary depending on the specific product and individual needs. It's important to follow the recommended dosage on the product label or consult with a healthcare professional for personalized guidance.

How to Use: Lymphalin capsules are typically taken orally with water, while liquid forms may be mixed with water or juice before consumption. It's often recommended to take Lymphalin on an empty stomach for optimal absorption.

Side Effects: Lymphalin is generally considered safe for most people when used as directed. However, some individuals may experience mild side effects such as gastrointestinal discomfort or allergic reactions to certain ingredients. It's important to consult with a healthcare provider before starting any new supplement regimen, especially if you have underlying health conditions or are taking medications.

Manjakani:

Definition: Manjakani, also known as Quercus infectoria or oak gall, is a natural substance derived from the oak tree. It has been used for centuries in traditional medicine for its potential health benefits, particularly for women's health and vaginal tightening.

Ingredients: Manjakani contains various bioactive compounds, including tannins, flavonoids, and gallic acid. These compounds are believed to contribute to the herb's medicinal properties, including its potential as an astringent and antiseptic agent.

How to Prepare: Manjakani is typically available in powder, capsule, or liquid extract form. It can be taken orally or used topically depending on the intended use. For vaginal tightening, manjakani may be applied topically as a gel or inserted into the vagina in capsule form.

Dosage: The appropriate dosage of manjakani can vary depending on factors such as age, health status, and the specific preparation being used. It's important to follow the recommended dosage on the product label or consult with a qualified herbalist or healthcare professional for personalized guidance.

How to Use: Manjakani can be taken orally or used topically depending on the intended use. It's important to use manjakani products as directed and to discontinue use if any adverse effects occur.

Side Effects: Manjakani is generally considered safe for most people when used in moderate amounts. However, some individuals may experience allergic reactions or skin irritation when used topically. It's important to use manjakani under the guidance of a healthcare professional and to discontinue use if any adverse effects occur.

Tila:

Definition: Tila, also known as linden flower or lime blossom, refers to the flowers of the Tilia genus, primarily Tilia europaea and Tilia cordata. These trees are native to Europe, but they are also cultivated in other regions for their fragrant and medicinal flowers.

Ingredients: Tila flowers contain various bioactive compounds, including flavonoids, phenolic acids, and volatile oils. These compounds are believed to contribute to the herb's medicinal properties, including its potential as a mild sedative, anxiolytic, and anti-inflammatory agent.

How to Prepare: Tila flowers are typically prepared and consumed as an herbal tea or infusion. To make tea, dried tila flowers are steeped in hot water for several minutes before being strained and consumed.

Dosage: The appropriate dosage of tila can vary depending on factors such as age, health status, and the specific preparation being used. It's important to follow the recommended dosage on the product label or consult with a qualified herbalist or healthcare professional for personalized guidance.

How to Use: Tila tea is typically taken orally. It's often consumed in the evening as a calming bedtime beverage or during times of stress or anxiety. It's important to use tila products as directed and to discontinue use if any adverse effects occur.

Side Effects: Tila is generally considered safe for most people when used in moderate amounts. However, some individuals may experience allergic reactions or digestive upset. It may also interact with certain medications or have adverse effects in individuals with certain health conditions. It's important to use tila under the guidance of a healthcare professional and to discontinue use if any adverse effects occur.

Red Clover:

Definition: Red clover, scientifically known as Trifolium pratense, is a flowering plant belonging to the legume family. It's native to Europe, Western Asia, and Northwest Africa but has been naturalized in many other regions. Red clover has been used in traditional medicine for various purposes, including its potential to support women's health and menopausal symptoms.

Ingredients: Red clover contains several bioactive compounds, including isoflavones (such as genistein and daidzein), flavonoids, and phytoestrogens. These compounds are believed to contribute to the herb's medicinal properties, including its potential as a hormone-balancing agent and its ability to support cardiovascular health.

How to Prepare: Red clover is typically prepared and consumed as an herbal tea or tincture. To make tea, dried red clover flowers are steeped in hot water for several minutes before being strained and consumed. Tinctures are prepared by steeping the flowers in alcohol or vinegar to extract their active compounds.

Dosage: The appropriate dosage of red clover can vary depending on factors such as age, health status, and the specific preparation being used. It's important to follow the recommended dosage on the product label or consult with a qualified herbalist or healthcare professional for personalized guidance.

How to Use: Red clover tea or tincture is typically taken orally. It's important to use red clover products as directed and to discontinue use if any adverse effects occur.

Side Effects: Red clover is generally considered safe for most people when used in moderate amounts. However, some individuals may experience allergic reactions or digestive upset. It may also interact with certain medications or have adverse effects in individuals with certain health conditions. It's important to use red clover under the guidance of a healthcare professional and to discontinue use if any adverse effects occur.

Sarsaparilla:

Definition: Sarsaparilla refers to several species of plants belonging to the Smilax genus, including Smilax regelii and Smilax officinalis. It has been used historically in traditional medicine for its potential health benefits, particularly for its purported detoxifying and anti-inflammatory properties.

Ingredients: Sarsaparilla contains various bioactive compounds, including saponins (such as sarsaponin and smilagenin), flavonoids, phenolic acids, and sterols. These compounds are believed to contribute to the herb's medicinal properties, including its potential as a diuretic, blood purifier, and anti-inflammatory agent.

How to Prepare: Sarsaparilla root is typically prepared and consumed as an herbal tea, decoction, or tincture. To make tea, dried sarsaparilla root is steeped in hot water for several minutes before being strained and consumed. Decoctions involve boiling the root in water to extract its active compounds, while tinctures are prepared by steeping the root in alcohol or vinegar.

Dosage: The appropriate dosage of sarsaparilla can vary depending on factors such as age, health status, and the specific preparation being used. It's important to follow the recommended dosage on the product label or consult with a qualified herbalist or healthcare professional for personalized guidance.

How to Use: Sarsaparilla tea or tincture is typically taken orally. It's important to use sarsaparilla products as directed and to discontinue use if any adverse effects occur.

Side Effects: Sarsaparilla is generally considered safe for most people when used in moderate amounts. However, some individuals may experience allergic reactions or digestive upset. It may also interact with certain medications or have adverse effects in individuals with certain health conditions. It's important to use sarsaparilla under the guidance of a healthcare professional and to discontinue use if any adverse effects occur.

Red Raspberry:

Definition: Red raspberry, scientifically known as Rubus idaeus, is a species of raspberry native to Europe and northern Asia. It's widely cultivated for its delicious berries and has been used in traditional medicine for various purposes, including its potential to support women's health during pregnancy and childbirth.

Ingredients: Red raspberry contains several bioactive compounds, including flavonoids, ellagic acid, anthocyanins, and vitamin C. These compounds are believed to contribute to the herb's medicinal properties, including its potential as an antioxidant, anti-inflammatory, and uterine tonic.

How to Prepare: Red raspberry leaf is typically prepared and consumed as an herbal tea or infusion. To make tea, dried red raspberry leaves are steeped in hot water for several minutes before being strained and consumed.

Dosage: The appropriate dosage of red raspberry leaf can vary depending on factors such as age, health status, and the specific preparation being used. It's important to follow the recommended dosage on the product label or consult with a qualified herbalist or healthcare professional for personalized guidance.

How to Use: Red raspberry leaf tea is typically taken orally. It's often recommended for pregnant individuals in the later stages of pregnancy to support uterine health and prepare for childbirth. It's important to use red raspberry leaf products as directed and to discontinue use if any adverse effects occur.

Side Effects: Red raspberry leaf is generally considered safe for most people when used in moderate amounts. However, some individuals may experience allergic reactions or digestive upset. Pregnant individuals should consult with a healthcare professional before using red raspberry leaf, especially if they have any underlying health conditions or are taking medications. It's important to use red raspberry leaf under the guidance of a healthcare professional and to discontinue use if any adverse effects occur.

Rhubarb:

Definition: Rhubarb, scientifically known as Rheum rhabarbarum, is a perennial plant cultivated for its edible stalks. While primarily used in culinary applications, rhubarb has also been utilized in traditional medicine for its potential health benefits, particularly for digestive health.

Ingredients: Rhubarb stalks contain various bioactive compounds, including anthraquinones (such as emodin and rhein), fiber, vitamins (such as vitamin K), and minerals (including calcium and potassium). These compounds are believed to contribute to the herb's medicinal properties, including its potential as a laxative and digestive aid.

How to Prepare: Rhubarb stalks are typically cooked before consumption, as the raw stalks are very tart and can be unpleasant to eat. They are often used in pies, crisps, jams, sauces, and other desserts, as well as in savory dishes. Rhubarb can also be used to make compotes, jams, and preserves.

Dosage: There is no specific dosage for rhubarb in culinary applications, as it is used as a food rather than a medicinal herb. However, when used for its potential laxative effects, it's important to consume rhubarb in moderation to avoid gastrointestinal upset.

How to Use: Rhubarb stalks can be chopped and cooked in various dishes, including pies, sauces, and jams. It's important to remove and discard the leaves, as they contain toxic compounds. When using rhubarb for its potential laxative effects, it's typically consumed as part of a cooked dish or in the form of a rhubarb-based herbal remedy.

Side Effects: Rhubarb stalks are generally safe for most people when consumed in moderate amounts as part of a balanced diet. However, excessive intake may lead to digestive upset or adverse effects due to the presence of oxalic acid, which can bind to calcium and form kidney stones in susceptible individuals. It's important to use rhubarb in moderation and to consult with a healthcare professional if you have any concerns or underlying health conditions.

Burdock:

Definition: Burdock, scientifically known as Arctium lappa, is a biennial plant native to Europe and Asia but now found worldwide. It's part of the Asteraceae family and has been used for centuries in traditional medicine and culinary practices.

Ingredients: Burdock contains various nutrients, including carbohydrates, fiber, vitamins (such as vitamin B6, folate, and vitamin C), and minerals (including potassium, magnesium, and manganese). It also contains active compounds such as polyphenols and volatile oils.

How to Prepare: Burdock can be prepared and consumed in various ways. The roots, leaves, and seeds are all utilized for different purposes. The root is commonly used in cooking, herbal teas, tinctures, and supplements, while the leaves and seeds are sometimes used in herbal preparations.

Dosage: The appropriate dosage of burdock root can vary depending on the specific form and intended use. For culinary purposes, there are no strict dosage guidelines, but for supplements or herbal remedies, it's essential to follow the recommended dosage on the product label or consult with a healthcare professional.

How to Use: Burdock root can be used in cooking by peeling, slicing, and adding it to soups, stews, stir-fries, or salads. It can also be brewed into a tea or used to make tinctures or extracts for medicinal purposes. Some people may also take burdock root supplements in capsule or powder form.

Side Effects: While burdock is generally considered safe for most people when consumed in moderate amounts, some individuals may experience allergic reactions or digestive upset. Additionally, burdock may interact with certain medications or have adverse effects in individuals with certain health conditions, such as diabetes or allergies to plants in the Asteraceae family. It's important to consult with a healthcare provider before using burdock, especially if you have underlying health conditions or are taking medications.

Cascara Sagrada:

Definition: Cascara Sagrada, scientifically known as Rhamnus purshiana, is a species of buckthorn native to western North America. It has been used traditionally as a laxative and to promote bowel regularity.

Ingredients: The primary active ingredients in cascara sagrada are anthraquinone glycosides, particularly cascarosides A and B. These compounds stimulate peristalsis in the colon, leading to increased bowel movements.

How to Prepare: Cascara sagrada is typically prepared as an herbal tea, tincture, or capsule. To make tea, dried cascara sagrada bark is steeped in hot water for several minutes before being strained and consumed. Tinctures are prepared by steeping the bark in alcohol to extract its active compounds.

Dosage: The appropriate dosage of cascara sagrada can vary depending on the specific preparation and intended use. It's important to follow the recommended dosage on the product label or consult with a healthcare professional for personalized guidance.

How to Use: Cascara sagrada tea or tincture is typically taken orally. It's important to start with a low dose and gradually increase if needed to avoid potential side effects such as cramping or diarrhea.

Side Effects: Cascara sagrada is considered safe for short-term use when used as directed. However, long-term or excessive use may lead to dependence, electrolyte imbalance, or dehydration. It may also interact with certain medications or have adverse effects in individuals with certain health conditions. It's important to use cascara sagrada under the guidance of a healthcare professional and to discontinue use if any adverse effects occur.

Cell Food:

Definition: Cell Food is a dietary supplement marketed as a highly oxygenating and alkalizing formula. It's claimed to support overall health and vitality by providing essential nutrients and oxygen to the cells.

Ingredients: The exact ingredients of Cell Food can vary depending on the brand, but it typically contains a proprietary blend of minerals, enzymes, electrolytes, and trace elements. Some common ingredients may include purified water, dissolved oxygen, seawater extract, and plant-based enzymes.

How to Prepare: Cell Food is usually available in liquid form and is typically taken orally. It can be consumed directly or diluted in water or juice before consumption.

Dosage: The dosage of Cell Food can vary depending on the specific product and individual needs. It's important to follow the recommended dosage on the product label or consult with a healthcare professional for personalized guidance.

How to Use: Cell Food is typically taken orally, either directly or mixed into water or juice. It's important to shake the bottle well before use and to store it according to the manufacturer's instructions.

Side Effects: Cell Food is generally considered safe for most people when used as directed. However, some individuals may experience mild digestive upset or allergic reactions to certain ingredients. It's essential to consult with a healthcare provider before starting any new supplement regimen, especially if you have underlying health conditions or are taking medications.

Chaparral:

Definition: Chaparral, scientifically known as Larrea tridentata, is a shrub native to the southwestern United States and northern Mexico. It has been used for centuries by Native American tribes for its medicinal properties and is commonly used in herbal medicine today.

Ingredients: Chaparral contains several bioactive compounds, including nordihydroguaiaretic acid (NDGA), flavonoids, lignans, and volatile oils. NDGA is believed to be the primary active compound responsible for many of chaparral's therapeutic effects.

How to Prepare: Chaparral can be prepared and consumed in various forms, including teas, tinctures, capsules, and topical preparations. To make tea, dried chaparral leaves are steeped in hot water for several minutes before being strained and consumed. Tinctures are prepared by steeping the herb in alcohol or vinegar to extract its active compounds.

Dosage: The appropriate dosage of chaparral can vary depending on the specific form and intended use. It's important to follow the recommended dosage on the product label or consult with a healthcare professional for personalized guidance.

How to Use: Chaparral tea or tincture is typically taken orally. It can also be applied topically to the skin for certain conditions. It's important to use chaparral products as directed and to discontinue use if any adverse effects occur.

Side Effects: Chaparral is generally considered safe for most people when used in moderate amounts. However, excessive intake or prolonged use may lead to liver toxicity or other adverse effects. It may also interact with certain medications or have adverse effects in individuals with certain health conditions. It's important to use chaparral under the guidance of a healthcare professional and to discontinue use if any adverse effects occur.

THE END